THREE FEET, THREE HOURS

ONE PHYSICIAN'S EXPERIENCE WITH ADDICTION AND RECOVERY

BY C. K. BREMEL, MD

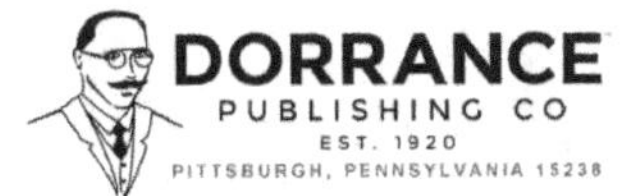

DORRANCE
PUBLISHING CO
EST. 1920
PITTSBURGH, PENNSYLVANIA 15238

Dorrance Publishing Co
585 Alpha Drive
Pittsburgh, PA 15238
Visit our website at *www.dorrancebookstore.com*

ISBN: 979-8-8872-9100-0
eISBN: 979-8-8872-9600-5

THREE FEET, THREE HOURS

ONE PHYSICIAN'S EXPERIENCE WITH ADDICTION AND RECOVERY

For all who suffer with addiction, and those that suffer along with them.

My utmost gratitude to all who have been so supportive on my journey:

My wife Kari, my children Ben, Rylee, Max, and Lucas for their unending love and tolerance.

Mike, Bruce, Sam, Kevin, and all of my friends.

My blessed Shoemaker brothers. Hutah!

And thank you eternally to Hazelden/Betty Ford Center for helping me out of the darkest days of my life and into a life of love and peace.

TABLE OF CONTENTS

INTRODUCTION

I am a board-certified physician who had a successful practice for twenty-seven years. Had, past tense. For the last eight years I have slowly but completely destroyed my life due to substance use, alcohol being the wrecking ball. I had a wonderful life, beautiful family, beautiful house, fancy cars, and my dream career. I had fun and caring friends with great camaraderie. I traveled, and I wanted for nothing. Or so I thought. It was only after I lost my family did I even start to wonder what was going on. I went to therapy, and AODA counseling for years. I went to AA and NA meetings off and on. I read and studied voraciously. Despite my efforts, I had only brief periods of sobriety. I became more and more baffled the more I learned, why couldn't I stop? Surely I could figure this out! For a while, I was convinced that I was completely normal and that I was a victim of the cold, cruel world. After all, I am a kind, loving, giving, and caring person. I was in and out of therapy from the age of seventeen, due to previous family turmoil, certainly all of that was handled by now. I was just reacting to my environment. But it took a long time to admit that it was something inside me that was driving the addiction, and subsequently driving everyone and everything away.

After all was lost, and legal issues and debt mounted, I sought treatment from a residential facility. I was finally able to track down my demons, confront them, and eliminate their power over me. I found that I had predispositions for addiction that I never dreamed of. As I have investigated, I found solid common themes in addicts and alcoholics. Shared evils of self-hatred and inadequacy, which resulted in ever-deepening isolation through experiences of humiliation and peculiarity, whether real or imagined. With an addict's psyche already developed into a canvas prepped with tremendous sensitivity, even sacrificial benevolence, the inability to handle rejection, usury, and even simple confrontation with maturity turn the addict inward for blame and self-destruction.

I offer my story, my experience and education, formal and informal, to all who wish to further understand addiction and alcoholism. I am compelled to relate my story to combat the existing prejudice toward addiction. Addiction is a mental illness. Addiction is a disease of the mind, body, and spirit. The brain is an organ of the body. It can malfunction, just like a kidney or heart or any other organ in the body. But addiction manifests itself as behavior. The behaviors are the symptoms of the disease. For millennia, addicts and others with mental illness have been ostracized, punished, beaten, imprisoned, even executed. Within the last several decades there has been improvement in understanding, but society as a whole judges mental illness symptoms as purposeful. This prejudice I harbored myself for most of my adult life. Many of my loved ones over these years have been saying "Why don't you just quit?" or "Pull your head out of your ass!" While not helpful to an addict, it demonstrates the prejudice I speak of. But I offer another approach. My question back is, "Do you truly believe one would purposely continue drinking/using for a high, just for fun, knowing the substance was taking everything from them?" Addictive behavior has little to do with the "high." Using, to an addict, becomes like breathing, a necessity for living. It stops being "fun" very early on. When the addict's brain experiences the numbing effect of the drug, this relief of spiritual pain quickly supplants reason. The numbing substance, the demon, sometimes referred to as "slick," or frequently more vernacular designations, hi-jacks the addict's brain and convinces the soul that it must do anything to get the numbing back. And as life goes on with the dysfunction in coping, along with a degree of tolerance, the more frequently and stronger the numbing needs to be. Hence the escalation of using.

In my darkest hours of addiction, I experienced tremendous desperation. I thought for sure that I was smart enough and loving enough to figure my way out of this horrible place. I remember sobbing on multiple occasions, so strongly that I could hardly breathe. I was so angry and hateful towards my own self. I would pray to God for some relief, some modicum of understanding of why I was behaving so irrationally. Sometimes the sobbing would come after I had been drinking, sometimes when I was completely sober. Usually within hours I was drinking again, continuing the insanity. Of course, this just builds self-hatred and violates any personal contract of trust or honesty. I cannot fathom a deeper desperation then complete lack of trust in oneself.

I am trying to inform and fight a prejudice that I have fully experienced myself. I am not here to garner pity or make excuses. I simply wish for understanding of addiction for all touched by this disease. I thank you all for your consideration. I do hope this is helpful to any who suffer, either directly or indirectly, from this horrible disease.

Peace.

1. THE EMPATH

His very first memory of childhood is somewhat nebulous. He was standing near the center of the living room. He was no more than two or three years old. The room was cool and damp, barely lit, as though a small candle illuminated the center, though no flame was apparent. The periphery blurred into gray. There was a hint of vanilla in the musty air. His mother was sitting cross-legged on the floor, rocking slowly and rhythmically back and forth, holding his crying sister. The mother was humming "Old Rugged Cross" while hypnotically yet dutifully soothing her child. She was staring straight ahead, seemingly entranced. The sister was about five years old; he was not sure why she was crying. Her sobbing upset him; he felt scared. He remembers approaching them, wanting only to be held by his mother. Without even a glance or other break in her stare, she somewhat robotically put her arm out and pushed him away. He stumbled slightly backwards against the couch behind him. He stood there and watched in bewilderment for what seemed like an eternity. Self-pity was thick in the surrounding air. At the time he did not, could not comprehend the parental need for Mom to comfort the sister. All he felt was entitlement and rejection admixed with confusion and resentment. He doesn't remember crying, but he probably did.

That toddler was me. I began my journey on the self-pity train at that time. I was ignorant of the import of this occurrence for so many years. Like many little ones at that age, I was very self-centered and attention seeking, requiring appropriate nurturing. The need for Mom's approval was paramount to obtaining that nurturing. With three older siblings, I suppose I was treated like a baby longer than most. I love my mother and father very much, and I am not here to throw them under the bus or shift blame. Like many parents in that era, they were children raising children. These stories from my life are meant only to illustrate and explain the psychological milieu which afforded development of addiction. As I pursued understanding of my undoing over these last years, I was surprised and enlightened at the commonalities of character, personality, and experiences shared by addicts and alcoholics. I discovered far more likenesses than differences.

I define the word empath here as a human with such extreme empathy as to closely identify with another's feelings or emotions. The word empath has also been used in science fiction to imply an element of paranormal mental telepathy. Here I simply invoke the extreme empathy definition, as it is used in ever-widening psychology circles.

When I was a little older, perhaps six or seven, my mom told me a story. She had suffered a tremendous loss; both of her parents were killed in a traffic accident when she was about three months pregnant with me. The physician told her she was going through too much and she should abort me in the interest of her own health. She tells the story that she slammed her fist on his desk and said, "No! I have lost too much already!" The doctor put my mother on valium to help with her grief. She was on that for years after as well (Mother's little helper). There was already the innate need in me for maternal approval; I propose it was stronger than most. Her story of fighting to keep me increased that need exponentially and cultivated a perverse sense of indebtedness.

I was raised in a midwestern Christian household, fostering an idealistic, superficial, and emotionally constrained, like many Christian households at the time. The golden rule was repeated time and time again, "Do unto others as you would have them do unto you." This became engrained in self, as well as the presumption and expectation of others. This was the beginning of creation of an extreme empath. The weight of the indebtedness I felt toward my mother was crushing. My mom was an only child, and my dad doted on her with fervent endeavors appreciated only dismissively. While she did what housewives did then, cook, clean, childcare etc., she also demonstrated extreme disappointment, in life, essentially. The family would take Sunday drives, only to have my mother point out all of the beautiful houses. While verbalizing awe there was an undertone of envy. The mantras that there are starving children in the world and that "there is always someone worse off than you" were repeated through the years.

I remember my first brand new truck, an opulent SUV. I was so proud of it as it was my first significant "reward" for medical school and residency, I called Mom. Once again seeking her approval. I was excited, silly, admittedly boastful, but I felt it warranted at the time, after all, one can only handle so much "delayed gratification" while living in this material world. I told her about the truck excitedly. Curiously, there was somewhat of a long pause. "I don't have a new truck… ?" she said softly, sounding bewildered.

I do not remember the rest of the conversation, just emptiness.

I started practicing medicine in 1995. I was very successful, and my patients were dedicated. Many of the nurses I worked with as well as other staff were extremely complimentary of my work; it always made me feel good when nurses and staff would tell me that I had the best bedside manner of any doctor they had ever worked with. I am very proud to say that I heard those words often.

I was brashly referred to as a "cash cow" by some administrators, due to my economic production that was rooted in a strong work ethic, a gift from my father. I was a hard worker from early childhood. Got a paper route as early as I could, then a busboy, gardener, fast food and auto parts. I was good out of the gate, employers/bosses loved me. But, in retrospect, I always seemed to have a huge ego build up fast. The entitlement for raises and recognition exploded with the "atta boy's." I could not understand why I was not being recognized financially if I was so good. The naivete and immaturity of unrealistic expectations cost me several jobs. The word immaturity has significant negative connotations; I prefer to use "incomplete self." We will explore this in greater detail later.

Doing more than what's expected can be a wonderful work ethic. I was taught that you go in early and stay late, and that there's no such thing as "That's not my job," to always do your best, and to help your coworkers when you can. It's best to not expect notice for that, don't perform good work for adulation or recognition. If you do go above and beyond, which is admirable, do not expect kudos. The most important pat on the back is the one you get from you. Other people who are truly grateful and will show gratitude for extra effort are few and far between. It's not like extra credit in school. I do not like being pessimistic; however, in my experience, going above and beyond demonstrates an easy mark, more frequently benefitting others than myself. Today, I do my best, then, to celebrate my work ethic as my victory. Another issue with expectations, as mentioned previously, is the development of resentments. Feelings of entitlement for unsolicited services and performance are completely undeserving. This was a long and hard lesson for me to learn. Now, I try to not even go down that path. I just try to do the next right thing, hopefully keeping any expectations in check.

The naivete of youth persisted, as I believed surely everyone had been taught the golden rule and was going to live by it. Obviously, the world does not work that way. The misguided trust and gullibility forged subsequent disappointment and feelings of betrayal. Consider what happens to a child while in the vulnerable and delicate development stages of personality, then add the duress of trauma or neglect. It is said Kaspar Hauser coined the term "soul murder." Efforts of the self, striving for identity, only to be awash in ambiguity and subjugation. The efforts to vet and adopt behavior were met with conflict and indecision. Trust was fragile and fleeting, resulting in prevalent and pervasive epistemic ambivalence. The behavior patterns were misshapen and subsequently delayed from lack of nurturing or direction. The frenetic result fostered misunderstanding and indecision. This effect was multiplied by reinforcement, the dependent reciprocity of learned behaviors. I attribute my social myopia to this phenomenon, that is my inability to "see the forest for the trees." Resultant personality traits and cognitive processing patterns were deemed indicative of attention deficit disorder and a degree of autism spectrum disorder according to mental health professionals.

Castigation and punishment were not terribly frequent during my childhood, but I had my share I suppose. Spankings were not frequent, just a "reminder." I admit several were severe enough that the wooden spoon or hairbrush broke, even a broom once. But never was medical attention required. Consequences of the transgression, but strangely, I don't remember the infractions. I do remember hearing the distant laughter of my parents and siblings after I was banished to my room. I could not understand how they could be laughing. How could they not feel any sympathy toward my suffering? I'm upset, they should be upset also. Now I understand life goes on; I was the one that screwed up, and they were not laughing at me. But at the time I extrapolated, multiplied, and exaggerated their seeming indifference to my anguish, further assailing my developing persona. I felt as though I had been excommunicated from the family, discarded as chaff. The feelings of isolation and alienation hurt more than the physical punishings. Later, the significance of the "spankings" was recorded by my treating health care professionals as physical abuse, not justifiable corrective corporal punishment.

The dichotomy of self-pity and near martyrdom develops with frank polarization. This sets up such conflict that there is nearly a dissociative aspect to the self. Enter Slick, the demon of addiction. Such a deep-seated sense of empathy coupled with essentially blind and misguided trust in others left me emotionally exposed and vulnerable. I was bullied relentlessly, incapable of gathering myself and exercising any instinctive defense, let alone one that was cogent. My Scandinavian roots caused me to flush easily, the red-faced stammering only inviting further ridicule. This advertisement of susceptibility has persisted my entire life. Apoplexy has always been my instinctive response, albeit undesirable, from the fight/flight/freeze reflex, so physical defense or altercation was out of the question. I found the idea of fighting abhorrent. I could never see myself purposefully harming another. I remember a few episodes of wrestling with friends, just messing around. I only did this a few times, as it seemed to me that every time I did, I wound up hurting the other person. While clearly unintentional and their injuries not serious, I still experienced such tremendous regret and shame that I would avoid any further sessions of "grab-ass." This caused further ostracization amongst the testosterone crowd, particularly in school and work settings. I admit that when my kids were of age for horsing around, I tried, but the trepidation won out, and these episodes were terribly sparse and brief. Worse yet, my kids seemed to sense my apprehension, and not understanding the source of my uneasiness they met my playfulness with fearful flinching and looks of distrust. I stopped immediately, of course, trying to restore loving and reassurance, desperate to conceal and assuage my anguish.

I identified with other victims of bullying, and many became very good friends from childhood. Our hearts had been broken and spirits were in tatters, as we suffered much of the same humiliation, and many of the same inequities. I comforted and cried with many of my friends at times. As I tried to mature and develop some sense of self, my empathy for the vulnerable and the resentments for bullies forged a disdain for "the cool kids." The kids with the expensive shoes, the latest styles, popularity, money, and family notoriety were regarded with condemnation by my friends and I for their bullying and teasing. I have never understood how any human being could get satisfaction, let alone entertainment, from another's misfortune and pain. It appeared to me the perpetrators somehow fed on the frustration and humiliation of others. I believe the gratification felt for another's adversity is misplaced ego fodder and has nefarious roots. Any delight shared by an aggressor is a flame fanned by mob mentality. The social glue actively reinforcing the behavior is the mortification of a common quarry.

Later in adulthood, I found myself generalizing and having a significant resentment toward not just popularity but simply attractive people as well. I have been outright laughed at, and that hurts enough, but the look of disgust from an attractive woman as she looked me up and down was soul crushing. In retrospect, I blame myself for giving them that power. I saw them get passes on mistakes, simply shown favor. Taller men, prettier women, all of the "beautiful people," going through life with doors flying open at their behest. The envy was pervasive and horrible. In my forties, as I examined my inventory of egregious behavior, I wound up despising myself even further for harboring such prejudice. Eventually, I realized much of the perceived favor they received was simply manifestation of my resentment.

Most of the resentment stemmed from my own inequities, mostly social awkwardness. As I said previously, bullying resulted, and frank ostracization. In my teens and twenties I learned I could charm many people out of the gate and do quite well initially, but I was soon floundering for any cohesive and acceptable personality traits. In all truthfulness I'm quite amazed that I did as well as I did in our society.

Regarding the observation of a dissociative aspect to the personality developing from this type of upbringing, I am convinced that this is how "Slick" came into existence, as noted above. Slick is a name given to the voice or force or demon that drives one to use. I have heard it used in many recovery circles. This demon of addiction develops from a culmination of factors. As noted in multiple studies, there is a heritable factor to addiction, but I have experienced and witnessed that the majority of the properties of addiction appear to be more from nurture than nature. There is extensive research currently in the area of trauma, and that is being looked at as a major factor for the development of addiction. Trauma is being defined as anything less than nurturing. The data is fleshing out the finding that the earlier the trauma, along with consideration for severity, the greater the risk for development of addiction.

2. IT'S NOT THEM, IT'S ME

What happens when you throw the empath into a sea of competition, greed, materialism, and selfishness? If the canvas is prepped with sensitivity and fragility as described above, the result is devastating. The empath may have enough intelligence to cope for years, but the conflict builds. In the early years, the resentments grow, the pervasive nature of the "good boy" morals soon had me turning inward for answers, such that surely they can't *all* be wrong, it must be something with me. With the infighting of the superego and the ID, the ego, that defender of self-esteem, is beat down. Self-hatred replaces self-preservation, and the unchecked/untreated result is the unconscious desire for death. For me it became the thought that it would be okay if I didn't wake up tomorrow. At one point, during my darkest hours, the only reason I would not commit suicide was that my family would miss out on a large life insurance policy payout, further injuring them by my actions. I am amazed at the number of addicts who have related similar experiences. I believe strongly that addiction's goal is to kill the addict.

This is where many espouse "Self-pity!" "oh poor baby," weakness, wallowing, sap, wuss…or worse. Most can overcome a degree of criticism, external as well as from within. It's the frequency and severity of that criticism that are brought into question. I was able to maintain enough sense of self that I could perform well in school…if I absolutely had to. I carried little self-assurance, let alone confidence, into my twenties. I was horrible at the locker room talk, camaraderie with the "boys" was minimal, and mostly repulsive to me. I persevered just enough to play a little sports, but never felt any significant sense of belonging.

I have always been giving, in action and material things as well. If a person was in need, I jumped at the opportunity to help. Whether material or time or muscle, I always felt so good being able to help. Again, do unto others. In school I am not sure if my "teacher's pet" approach was from this desire to help or from attention seeking. I do remember the pernicious contempt from my classmates for my volunteerism, and I was left anticipating further retribution. Still embracing the need for approval and still seeking authoritative adulation I persisted, to my detriment socially. Later in life, I was a huge tipper. I would even give the oil change guys an extra hundred bucks when I got my oil changed! I remember giving each of the guys that installed my pool two hundred bucks each as a tip! I was always in an excited and impulsive state when I was so generous. When I would do such, I always heard the same thing from them, "Are you sure?" That made me smile too, because it was clear that they were surprised by it. Occasionally, I would be told "You don't have to do that." My response was always "That's why I do it!" I felt I was just sharing for my good fortune and paying it forward at the same time. I am sure there was some unconscious reciprocity here trying to repay God for my life and privilege, stuck in the "I owe others for my life." Whatever the impetus, giving always felt good.

I was the poster child for the "Nice guys finish last!" society. I tried to convince myself that that is what Christ would want me to do, and though I am still a firm believer in the Christian faith, my approach at that time was guileless and unworldly. I don't think Jesus was unhappy about my behavior, but so many aspects of earthly culture and society were adversarial, and with my faulty defense mechanisms, I was discarded and confined to a narrow existence of "assembling the widgets." I must admit that, for the most part, I found the factory floor comfortable, as I had become terrified of confrontation no matter how minor.

In the corporate and management world, I was deemed "not a team player." Probably because I never understood the game. I bristled at injustice, I joined others' fights and defended the working underdogs. My inability to effectively communicate during heightened emotions always ended in further ostracization and even reprimands. The perfect example was turf wars with medical colleagues. As usual, it was all about the almighty dollar. I remember working for minimum wage, my mind stuck on my sweating for others' gain. So juvenile entitlement and indignation persisted, righteousness presumed, prejudices growing.

I remember my grandmother prophetically espousing the axioms "The worst thing you can do is make a poor man rich" and "A fool and his money are soon parted." I was severely afflicted with the love of money, said to be the root of all evil. I was so focused on material things, the mimetic desires. No doubt that was me. Yes, spending was horrible, part of my addictive behavior, and my excessive generosity drove my wife nuts. The empath inside knew he could please others with gifts of materialistic and/or monetary gain. Gambling took over six figures from me. I understand that gambling itself is part of my addiction, but my tipping was more extravagant. My purchases were always top shelf, all of the amenities and appointments. Big luxury SUVs or even limos, as well as fancy hotel suites, were the accommodations when traveling with the family. I did not even argue about the price of a car. I felt nauseated and embarrassed bargaining. I was always a spendthrift, chasing the mimetic desires. I would buy an ATV or snowmobile, for instance, paying top dollar, bring it home for the "Oohs" and "Aahs," ride it a couple of times, and share it with the family, but soon, it just sat there. Then I would turn around and sell it at a substantial loss. Mostly because I just wanted to get rid of it (also at the behest of my irritated but patient spouse!). I admit I got joy out of seeing the elation in the buyer at getting such a great deal. I find it interesting that my reaction is completely opposite of most, who would, naturally, be upset at the loss. I experienced no such regret. Grandma was right about this fool!

Hence my personal battle within. From both nature and nurture I was blessed with wonderful qualities. I was forged and conditioned to be polite, friendly, and kind, the makings of a people pleaser. I was gregarious and amusing, loving to see laughter. Literally a "Good time Charlie." I treated everyone as a friend, a close friend, way too quick to trust. In review, I see that I was too trusting, gullible; one of my experienced counselors said I had a poorly functioning "shit detector." I have always had difficulty seeing the forest for the trees, burdened with a significant deficiency of common sense. This led to further feelings of alienation as I witnessed so many of my "friends" whispering and laughing furtively. I would like to say that those scenarios no longer happen, or that they don't bother me. But I cannot assert either. All of this just causing more shame.

Over these last years it has become apparent that my inappropriate social interactions stemmed from these traits of arrested emotional maturation. My social clumsiness exposed vulnerability, a significant chink in the armor during the developing years. But God bless Brené Brown. She elegantly explains how vulnerability is viewed as weakness by society's standards. Then she goes on to demonstrate that if you are honest and open, that takes courage, to be vulnerable. They are not opposites. I can appreciate this now. I have heard stories of addicts walking into the boss's office or approaching a spouse or family, saying one needed help. In allowing the desperation to manifest, and not shrug it off as though "It will be better tomorrow," the addict demonstrates tremendous vulnerability and courage. I believe this to be the nidus for surrender and proclaiming powerlessness. This opens the door for the acceptance for direction out of the morass of shame and self-pity built up over time. I have witnessed this self-loathing and self-hatred destroy lives and people, myself included. That's addiction. The tremendous isolation and feelings of undesirable uniqueness further strengthened desire for, and attempts at, acceptance by others, particularly caregivers. I have discussed the idea that perhaps there is purposeful acting out, essentially desiring being found out or caught. These discussions are very brief and never welcomed by whom I'm discussing it with. This stands to reason, as the premise is quite uncomfortable. I believe this occurs at an unconscious level, somewhat covertly learned through the younger years, again to assuage the desperate yearning for connection. I suppose there may be some who experienced conscious design, but I'm very skeptical, perhaps early in life. This would depend on how severe the emotional immaturity was. Later, as addiction takes hold and loss and trouble ensue, it is virtually impossible for me to imagine any conscious or purposeful involvement. But I entertained the idea that even negative attention *is* attention, although not likely to culminate in acceptance. In fact, sabotage of this goal would certainly be the result. Just more self-destructive behavior for an addict.

3. SELF

As an empath I was always looking to please people. Gaining their approval was of utmost importance, what I felt was the cornerstone of myself, my identity. If I could not please someone or were unable to win their approval, I was not reassured of the identity that my mind had created. The identity I had created was a superficial and tacit one. I reveled in others' delight and felt shameful and humiliated with their disappointment. I have felt tremendous sadness for those less fortunate. Even driving by a home in disarray and all kinds of junk in the yard, I felt despair and powerlessness. I felt very bad that I could not help those people. Part of me wished for a huge financial windfall so I could offer to help. I used to drive quite a bit, so I would see these places frequently; over the last six to eight years, this became more pronounced. When I drive past some garbage on the road, I feel compelled to stop and pick it up, and frequently have. I have even felt grief and sorrow for an animal lying dead on the side of the road. My mind would also go to the "grief" experienced by the animal's family, for lack of a better term. Arguably consequential, these examples drive home a point. My sense of owing my life to others had manifested completely.

Along with identity comes emotional maturity, to know how to react properly. That is to say the ability to react within reasonable social constructs and expectations. Of course, an entirely different subject matter is whether one is equipped with cognitive processing that can recognize, define, and respond to these constructs and expectations. Such is the case with mental health disorders such as depression or anxiety, autism, cognitive delay, and psychosis among others. When this maturation doesn't happen, one is not able to define oneself. How I react to an emotion demonstrates a portion of my personality. If I don't react as one would say "appropriately," that is within the constructs and expectations as described above, and appear cogent, then I will be dismissed by others and ineffective at defending myself. The best example for my inappropriate reactions or responses has to do with anger. While other emotions could also disarm me, my anger reaction was the most pronounced. I call it my "pufferfish" reaction. It is immediate and problematic. I was not violent, but red-faced and stammering for sure. I have found this pattern to be nearly ubiquitous amongst addicts. Diagnoses of attention deficit disorder, depression, anxiety, bipolar disease, and autism are just a few culpable conditions putting a human at markedly increased risk for developing addiction.

This is my goal here, as stated previously, education/information on the disease model for addiction. I hope to provide a modicum of clarity to these constructs and expectations that are so pervasive within our society. It is my most sincere hope to save other addicts some of the pain of this stigma that is attached to addiction in our world.

4. THE DISEASE

Many of us are investigating the disease of addiction because of pain. I know I have experienced and caused tremendous pain and will continue to study this disease for the rest of my days. Any addict or alcoholic that I have discussed this with has described horrific pain. Much of the pain seems to come from loss, particularly of family and friends/relationships but also of material things. There is also the pain of the legal ramifications of using. I believe some understanding can assuage that pain. Maybe we have a family member that is suffering from addiction or alcoholism. I'm going to say addiction to make things flow a little better. I will also use the terms "using" and "drinking" interchangeably. But we're all here because of pain from addiction. Addiction affects everyone the addict interacts with and is considered a "family disease" in most therapy circles.

Starting in the 1950s, the American Medical Association and other health authorities defined addiction as a disease. Many other authorities followed, to include the Centers for Disease Control and Prevention, the World Health Organization, and even the Centers for Medicare and Medicaid Services. This position has only been strengthened over the years. There are ICD-10 codes and even criteria for disability from this disease. The scientific evidence for addiction as a disease is clear and concise, and overwhelming. The major obstacle to acceptance of this concept is no different than racial prejudice. While racism is certainly a hot button topic, the premise behind it is simple. The simplest and most glaring fault of racism is hatred. Much of this hatred, if not all in this era, is learned. This is true of prejudice towards addicts as well. Just as some of the hatred may be aimed at various melatonin levels, so can it be directed toward unconventional behavior. Certainly, there is no disease process associated with skin color as presented, but the hateful treatment of both addiction and otherwise "different appearance" is similar, albeit arguably and imprecisely disproportionate. What remains is a contempt for the addict's perceived laziness and desire for debauchery.

The brain is simply an organ. As true with any organ systems of the body, there can be dysfunction. The major difference with brain dys-function is that it directly impacts social interaction through the be-havior of those afflicted. With humans being the social animals that we are, the behavior of the addict is seen as abhorrent. It is this lack of un-derstanding that fuels the judgment and disdain. The latest technology with respect to imaging has shown significant differences in functional and metabolic patterns of different areas of the brain when comparing addicts and non-addicts. The ability of science to measure this meta-bolic activity and neurotransmitter function has advanced significantly in the last several decades. Magnetic resonance imaging has provided tremendous insight into brain structure and function, in particular with development of the newer functional MRI process.

I will not reiterate all of the neuroscience that has been elucidated over the decades. The data is well recorded and available. The majority is readily available online. There is copious and scientifically rigorous objective data to support the disease model. It is no longer simply pa-tient interviews or surveys or hormonal blood levels. We can now ac-tually see and demonstrate the differences between the brains of the addict and non-addict. The findings of the neurotransmitter research have been extremely helpful in understanding further the changes in cognitive processing of the addict's mind. I direct the reader to the short documentary film entitled *Pleasure Unwoven*. The film is very concise in explaining these physiological changes, though becoming somewhat dated. From my own perspective, I don't necessarily agree with the title of the show, but I certainly agree with the premise. Perhaps when I was younger using/drinking was for pleasure, for social purposes.

When my drinking/using was at its worst from 2016 to 2021, I was certainly not drinking for pleasure. I was drinking alone; I did not want to be around anyone; the only purpose of the alcohol was to numb my pain and horrible thoughts. This strategy worked quite well for several years. Again, as my disease progressed, I lost more and more of my life. There is a common view in society that addicts and alcoholics simply want to be high all the time. The view is that there is significant immaturity, lack of responsibility and control, selfishness, apathy, and the desire to continue the high. These traits are certainly apparent when observing the behavior of the addict. I freely admit to many of these traits as above. Over the years of treatment, I have discovered the root of addiction is much deeper and much more complex. While it has been proven that the addict's brain tends to function differently, it has become clear that this difference, and subsequently the genetic propensity, is merely a risk factor. Not all people with these differences in cognitive function manifest addiction.

Addiction can manifest in multiple ways. The more recent term used for addiction is "substance use disorder." This nomenclature may be helpful for some aspects of treatment but does not include many others who suffer with addiction by means other than substance use. Other well described behaviors that follow the addiction pattern include gambling, overeating, sex addiction, spending and even exercise. If these behaviors are severe enough, they most certainly can destroy one's life. Interestingly, I find some of my scientific colleagues following a similar pattern of judgment and prejudice by parsing out what may be thought of as less dangerous manifestations of addiction. I have witnessed all types of addictive behavior destroy lives.

5. THE HIGHER POWER

I believe that one of the most important confessions that an addict can make is to say that they are imperfect. That does not sound too hard for most. Many times I have encountered those who have a very difficult time with the concept of a higher power. One of my questions to those that are struggling with this concept is, "Do you think or feel that you are perfect?" and of course, I have always heard "No" for their response. I further posit that if they are imperfect, it is logical to believe that perfection exists. Furthermore, I propose that a modicum of perfection exists in each of us. With this dialogue I have frequently witnessed addicts deep in thought after. I believe very strongly that perfection exists, and for me, that perfection is my higher power. But that is just my belief. Maybe it is entropy, for those minimalists out there. Entropy would be your answer because it is a natural law of physics stating that everything goes from order to disorder. So perhaps the entire universe over the next trillions of years will turn into nothing but a big ball of dust. That's what all the math leads to. Once again, scientific empirical data and laws of physics support this.

Another question that I have asked at the meetings is, "Are you grateful?" Of course, their answer is always a resounding "Yes." Then I follow with "What are you grateful for?" Then I usually hear things like, "I'm grateful that I got my cavity filled! It doesn't hurt anymore." I ask them to back up and tell me what they are really grateful for, dig deeper. Subsequently, pensively, they reply similar to "I'm grateful for my kids, my family, and the love I get from them. And I'm grateful that I have four limbs, and I'm grateful that I have a working brain and I have food and clothing and a roof over my head…" and I just about tear up because this is a very promising sign for an addict. I frequently hear wonderful and truthful gratitude. Then I ask them, "So that is what you are grateful for, now tell me who you are grateful *to*?" "If you're grateful for all these wonderful things, who or what are you grateful to?" This may stump them for a bit, but the idea of a higher power may be tacitly entertained.

Even if there is difficulty naming the phenomenon it may be a place to begin for understanding. Need a name? Pick one. It could be God. The word God can stand for the traditional view of an all-powerful being, or God could stand for group of drunks, or good, orderly direction. Other names to consider are Allah, Zeus, or Buddha; there are many. I will use the word God for brevity. The point of all of this is to accept a new paradigm for the self. A paradigm of imperfection, of gratitude, of vulnerability. Once I admitted that there is something more powerful than me, once I started to truly believe it, I was able to yield control. I was able to accept my imperfections, even embrace them. I did not have to be all powerful, nor could I be. Enter surrender. As my understanding grew, so did my peace and serenity. There is a saying in Alcoholics Anonymous that we can only keep what we have by giving it away. Specifically, I believe this means sobriety. I believe that to listen and share with another addict is giving of the self, validation of one's humanity, which in turn nourishes the spirit.

I'm a Christian. I have been since childhood. I was raised in a Protestant household. Occasionally churchgoing. I admit that in my teens and later I seldom went to church or prayed or read the Bible. My wife was quite diligent with our family with respect to Sunday school and church, and we attended important services for baptism and communion and holidays. I have always maintained my faith though certainly it waned. Demands of the material world interfering. After studying, meditating, and praying, I do feel a significantly renewed faith and feel very blessed and grateful for this. I do not believe God's "up there" pushing buttons and pulling levers and directing things. I believe God resides in all of us. I don't have any other explanation for that wonderful, joyous feeling I get at the meetings. I refuse to call it mob mentality or some other phrase that would suggest cult behavior. I believe it to be the higher power magnified by the collective soul of the group. Many of the people I have talked to had difficulty with the idea of divinity. I propose that there exists a bit of the higher power in each of us. That bit is, in and of itself, divine. I believe human is divine. I am met with quizzical looks from many addicts regarding this view, yet there is a hint of satisfaction. Giving up the need to control everything, to be everything, to have everything has been the greatest gift of salvation from my higher power resulting in my recovery.

There are also some very interesting scientific theories, particularly in the field of quantum mechanics and other perseverations of physics, philosophy, and theology. Some theories have posited that we are all figments in a dream of some higher order being. Or perhaps we are holograms in a certain dimension, a dimension amongst many dimensions. In any case we somehow were given an opportunity to exist. If we can accept the existence of this intelligence or being, then we can surrender and develop trust. As an addict, I had a tremendous problem with trust, even trusting myself. A very frightening place to be. I heard this from many addicts. But my trust in a higher power allowed me to let go of my need to control. I could take a deep breath and completely surrender to my higher power. Surrendering, accepting; these are powerful words for the self to achieve peace. Surrendering control is not giving up; it is the act of accepting life on life's terms. The best example I can give is that of discarding the need for favorable resolution. Yielding fate to the moment, where the higher power is. God is not in the past or the future, and it is a waste of time contemplating same. The concept that I am in charge waned. I did not have to dwell on my previous mistakes and resentments. The AA step two provides "We came to believe in a power greater than ourselves that could restore us to sanity," and that's exactly what I'm trying to describe here. I needed to surrender to that power; it just means I quit fighting, I quit trying to control, I had to quit trying to be my own higher power. So define your higher power however you like. Include the capacity for love, the kind of love you would have for your children, that being unwavering and unconditional. Perhaps a kinder word than surrender would be acceptance. Acceptance of peace, of the moment, of the self as is to include self-love, and of trust in a higher power. And acceptance of love, from your higher power as well as others. Love, like faith, is empty without works. You get out what you put in. A very distressing finding during my studies of addiction and recovery is the difficulty addicts have in confessing self-love. That certainly was an issue for me. The only path to self-love is through all the garbage. What is needed is acknowledging, defining, and subsequently discarding, to the extent possible, the self-hatred and self-loathing, the shame and the guilt. I was left with the thought that if I could not love myself, then how could I expect anyone else to? Purge the shame! Forgive unconditionally all who have wronged you, especially yourself! This allows you to love yourself, and truly love others.

6. LOVE

I must admit that I use the word love quite a bit. I consider love to be the source for recovery. So many friends have told me that while using heavily, they felt that they were not lovable. Many times, this circled back to childhood or adolescent trauma. Listening to addicts, it appears clear to me, and sensibly so, that the sooner the trauma happens in life, notwithstanding the degree of the trauma itself, the worse the damage. Sometimes it was exacerbated by adult trauma. My concept of my higher power, that being God, provides for a little bit of that power in each of us. While truly cliché, it works very well for what I am trying to describe. I consider God to be a light brighter than the sun, and each of us has some of that light within us. It is one of the best ways I know to describe the wonderful feeling I get at recovery meetings. I have shared this feeling at many meetings and have had other addicts share similar stories. All of those little "A-ha!" moments in the meetings when I feel like I'm being lifted up, like a weight is taken off of my shoulders, as though the light inside me gets brighter. I firmly believe that this light, this modicum of a higher power, this love, is what connects us all. I also believe that the absence of this light, meaning the absence of this love, indicates lack of connection. Brene Brown describes this beautifully. She discusses this need for connection. That is to say, the opposite of addiction is not sobriety or recovery but connection. As an optimist, I do not believe that there can be absence of this inner light, but certainly some have more firm connection than others.

My experience and education tell me that addiction wants to get me alone, wants me to isolate, and I experienced this firsthand for many years. Addiction is frequently referred to as a disease of shortage, lack, and insufficiency. Very true, for it is the loss of family and friends, even the job and its connections that perpetuate the isolation and lack of connection. Many may view my outlook on love and connection as being rather "pie in the sky" or auspicious. But I believe that to truly understand addiction one must first understand the process by which the addict becomes so isolated. Again, we are reminded of the lack of self, the presence of self-hatred, the buildup of egregious resentments resultant of overreaching efforts such as hard work and generosity, all culminating in the need for anesthesia through using. Subsequently, the more substance used the more self-flagellation and the deeper the depression, self-hatred increasing exponentially. Such a nasty view of oneself supports the attitude of believing others' rejection. Quite a horrific cycle, leading to "jails, institutions, and death." Plainly put, the addict requires love to heal. The treatment for addiction is love. In this context, love *is* the higher power, love is relationship and connection, love is human. With enough love and time, the goal of self-love for the addict can be achieved.

I have mentioned the joyous feeling I get at meetings, echoed by many addicts. I have noticed that this wonderful feeling is even more pronounced as the sharing gets deeper, and emotions run higher. Again, we can only keep what we have by giving it away, and I believe this to mean love as well. I believe that light of the higher power in each of us glows ever brighter as we share more, as we listen more. I have witnessed myself, and heard other addicts report that this light, when it burns ever brighter, is able to carry one through days in a more positive mindset. I sense it carrying me through difficult times. Therefore, I believe the meetings are so important for those in recovery. Sharing from the heart is key to an inspirational and restorative encounter. In the beginning you need to fill up your tank, your spiritual tank, but even later in recovery you need the occasional top-off. The best part about the love from God is that you don't have to go looking for it. Be honest, open minded, and willing to do the next right thing and you will find love and grace given to you freely. To maintain a robust recovery program, the relationships, connections, and love all require regular maintenance. The nature of the maintenance may simply be a phone call to reaffirm a relationship or connection, or it may simply be a prayer or meditation to feed the light.

I have reported social awkwardness and poor defensive skills. Of course, looking through the retrospectroscope, the ideas of autism spectrum disorder and other mental health issues are entertained as having a degree of culpability. Nevertheless, the alienation and fragility that resulted only worsened my social behavior. I offer an example regarding the use of "big words." If I am having a conversation and someone uses a word I do not understand, I may ask for clarification, but I'm certainly not going to tell someone that "nobody understands that word." That's not true. Many do know. My response is to look it up. In fact, it's my responsibility to look it up and educate myself. Again, isn't that what your grade schoolteacher told you to do? My colleagues are people with broad vocabularies. They use "big words." I'm not going to dumb things down, I think that's insulting. My purpose is to communicate effectively and cogently, which includes using the proper terms. The example of the problem is that I had another health care provider castigate me in the in the middle of the ER, in front of all my nurses and staff, literally yell, "No one knows what that means!" It was the word irascible, which simply means difficult, easily angered. Instead of using judgmental terms, irascible is more descriptive of a mood or state of mind. Maybe they don't feel good, maybe they're just acting out and being crabby because they're having problems. It's a neutral and nonjudgmental term. Rather than an insult, irascible defines just a temporary state of mind as being negative. So, I am simply being me, and yet I'm looked at as being conceited. During this exchange, because I am who I am, I did not respond. I could have easily told them to look it up. But given the circumstances in the emergency room, all the staff, and my lack of ability for articulation of arguments, I said absolutely nothing. Even though this seems terribly minor, the degree of sensitivity an empath possesses should be evident. I internalized the pejorative statement further assailing my spirit. This illustrates the process of self-destruction I outlined, how such a minor occurrence can inflict such a cascade of pain. Again I feel the need to reassert; please, no pity, I do not mean to make excuses. I am simply in the process of offering an explanation for addictive behavior. I have heard many addicts report minor issues such as this causing them disproportionally exaggerated emotions, and subsequently inappropriate reactions.

Sharing these seemingly innocuous stories at meetings has been very helpful, as there is usually some degree of agreement and identification from others. This is extremely helpful for that sense of belonging that addicts so desperately need. I found that the more I shared at the meetings the better I felt. It's like a weight being lifted. Deeper connection seems to be formed so much more by shared pain than shared pleasure. It is through identification with other addicts' pain on that divine human level that feeds the relationship. The old adage that misery loves company may be applicable here, but I prefer to use the term enlightenment.

Another example of the empath-indignation dichotomy is when I was in medical school. I did my obstetric training in a very busy obstetric unit. I saw such wonderful human beings giving birth, and what a beautiful thing that was. The patient and her significant other or coach, the resident, a nurse, and I were the five people in the room, but all of a sudden, there were six!

There was a senior resident that was not very pleased with me. I'm not sure why. I wrote good notes, I followed the patients well, the other residents seemed to think that I was doing a good job. My first labor patient was a lovely young lady giving birth to her second child. It was to be a normal vaginal delivery, nothing risky, but of course, she had to undergo labor. She experienced what I imagined were the expected pains and usual labor, and she successfully gave birth to the child without complication. She had to work very hard and was rewarded with a miracle. I was overwhelmed by the whole experience. I told the patient that I thought she was a hero and that I wasn't sure that I could have ever done that. The patient smiled, but the senior resident in question said, "I'm gonna make sure you get kicked off this service," right there in the delivery room in front of the patient, coach, and staff. Luckily, that resident was unsuccessful, and several of the other residents were very supportive of my approach. I suppose as an obstetric resident, surgical resident, she saw the weakness as something undesirable in the delivery room. And perhaps it was a show of some immaturity to verbalize my feelings, but I remember that patient and I having a wonderful rapport and hugging and shedding tears together. I'm glad I didn't let that experience change my approach to patients, because over the years I have shed tears and hugged an awful lot of my patients. I consider that the most rewarding aspect of my career. Again, connections made, however brief they may be.

7. HOPE

A side note on hope. Many people consider hope a significant part of faith. I believe hope to be an integral part of life, as it can offer solace when things aren't going particularly well, and it can offer light to a desire. Hope is something that you pray will guide you along the path that God has designed. Ancient mythology speaks of Pandora's box. When the box (original mythology, Greek, the box was actually a jar) was opened by her husband, all of the evils of the world escaped except for one, and that was hope. I have a difficult time considering hope an evil. I can understand the premise, as it does require you to live somewhat in the future. By doing so, one could lose necessary drive to achieve. One can also see hope as a type of fantasy or fantasizing. Fantasizing, to a certain degree, is considered characteristic of addiction. I propose that the difference between hope and fantasy is quite the chasm. Hope has more of a personal need implied whereas fantasy is likely to be pining after mimetic desires, "keeping up with the Jones'," and "desires of the flesh" shall we say. My approach is to stay out of the future as much as possible and to stay out of the past as well. I try very hard to stay in the moment. This spares me a trip down expectation lane to possible disappointment or resentment.

8. THREE FEET, THREE HOURS

After all of my experience in rehab and twelve-step programs, I am at peace with my approach. I have had to accept myself as I am. I am...

An empath, a dire one at that.
Extreme emotional sensitivity.
Intelligent but lacking common sense.
Not being able to see the forest for the trees.
Unwarranted and premature trust in others.
Lack of trust in self.
Generous to a fault.
Hard working.
An addict.

I have described the factors involved in my addiction to the best of my ability. I have witnessed many of these traits shared by other addicts who are suffering. While I am hoping that my story and information are helpful to addicts and their families, I wish to offer a brief strategy that has worked well for me. As I pointed out earlier, many of my problems stemmed from lack of emotional maturity, causing me to react without processing. Emotions are inescapable, natural, human. It is the reaction to emotion where we can have impact on how that emotion will affect our lives. The lessons of mindfulness, processing the moment, and understanding your responses to environmental stimuli are necessary for harmonious living. I offer these simple considerations during times of confusion, duress, or simple restlessness.

I notice if I'm daydreaming or bored it is easy to refocus, increase my awareness and perhaps my effectiveness. At these times the most difficult part is recognizing the loss of focus. More importantly, when the straying is abrupt, such as with an intrusive emotion, frequently to some external stimulus, I **pause** to acknowledge the distraction and refocus on that moment. The goal is to stay in the moment, as that is the only place I have any power. I have seen many examples of what "PAUSE" can stand for; I offer the following, which is blended from my experience.

Pause

Assess

Understand

Surroundings

Execute

<u>Pause</u> is exactly that, a pause, a deep breath as you evaluate what has happened to gain your attention.

<u>Assess</u> the reason for the distraction. Identify the emotions associated. Is this a true emergent situation?

<u>Understand</u> the cause for the emotion and draw from previous experience and education to calm yourself and process necessity and nature of a response.

<u>Surroundings</u> need to be taken into consideration. Is this the right time and place to react? Do I need to respond to this person in a more private setting?

<u>Execute</u> your response maturely, at a time when you can do so cogently and effectively. Too rapid or too emotional of a response is judged harshly.

I find this strategy to be very effective in bringing me back to the moment. I work hard to be present in the moment, as I do believe that's where God is. He is not in the past or the future, so I try not to spend my time there. This is a pragmatic approach for life in our material world, as, again, the present is the only place we have power.

I look at the ***three feet*** around me on a regular basis to see if there is anything I need to do right now. By focusing on my immediate surroundings, I can't help but be drawn back to the moment. I can refocus on the task at hand or process what is happening and ascertain whether I need respond at all. I have always said that when you don't feel normal you must do something normal. Get busy with your hands, wash the dishes, do some laundry, vacuum the rug. Anything to get some physical activity involved. This helps tremendously with focus and affords time to process whatever might be making you feel abnormal. I have found this very useful because even after a couple of minutes, I see the dishes are done, and I have been able to refocus. It is amazing at what completing a small task can do for you in the moment. Hobbies are quite effective in this role. Woodworking, knitting, quilting, puzzles or games can all be great at helping focus.

This process of mindfulness in the moment has been extremely helpful to me. The goal of PAUSE is at the core of cognitive behavioral therapy and dialectic behavioral therapy. There are many strategies to achieve awareness of the moment. I have found simple gratitude to be very centering and grounding. It's difficult to be sad or upset while you're counting your blessings. When I recognize a period of distraction that I feel is unnecessary or negative and I want to ground myself or recenter myself, I simply start thinking of all the things that I am grateful for. Again, these do not have to be huge things in your life, in fact I find the most satisfying are in a long list of little things. Meditation is helpful with this as well. Sometimes this is difficult, as I find meditation requires significant solace and quiet. This is not always attainable. But when I do have just a few minutes of calm, I can sit back comfortably in my chair with my hands on my knees, my legs uncrossed, and breathe in and out slowly. I count my breaths. I find it helpful to recite a poem or a song in my mind with frequent breaks of calm breathing.

As I look around, we are only talking about a six-foot circle, so it should not be terribly daunting. If there is a small task that needs to be done, then I can certainly go ahead and do it. But if it's just a matter of refocusing because my mind has wandered, that may be all I need to do, and that may take only a split second. If I find that that six-foot area is simply overwhelming, then the important process is to further calm down, I take more slow, deep breaths, even meditate for a bit if time allows. I can then decide if I want to do even a small part of what needs to be done, or perhaps I need to relocate or direct my attention elsewhere. Most of the time I can come back to it later. There is very little in life that is a crisis. Addicts are renowned for living crisis to crisis. Unfortunately, those crises are usually caused or even manufactured by us, the addict. The point of this exercise is simply mindfulness, refocusing to the moment, getting out of your head when you feel overwhelmed. These are the times you may be at risk for relapse, and it is very important to have a strategy in place for when you're feeling restless, irritable, or discontent. If this approach is interesting to you, I highly recommend reading more about mindfulness and cognitive behavioral therapy. You may also find significant insight from dialectic behavioral therapy.

The next strategy has to do with one day at a time. My approach is to focus on the moment, staying in the moment, as above. I have had times when I found myself needing to refocus quite frequently, when there is obviously a more complex environment. I can use the three feet strategy to refocus, but I admit there are times when the difficulties seem to be lasting longer. It is then that I begin to look at a longer period of time, specifically *three hours*, as that can break the day up nicely and provide some semblance of peace and relief. I look at the day as three or four periods of three hours each, being basically divided by mealtimes. I simply tell myself that it's only three hours, whether in the morning, or in the afternoon from after lunch to dinner time, or it may be the evening from dinner to bed. My design is simply to reduce the perceived enormity of the difficulty. I feel this makes it much easier to handle. By the way, when was the last time you took a "long lunch," or a day truly "off"? I have found that these little gestures of self-care are key for grounding. Addicts are at risk for relapse if they are over-whelmed. This is especially true of those in early recovery. Logic follows that the desired multitasking of our era is dangerous for those suffering from addiction. I also see this in those diagnosed with bipolar disease. The rapid, labile, and severe emotional reactions of bipolar disease are easily exacerbated by feelings of overload. Depression and anxiety, which frequently go hand in hand, are also worsened by the demands of multitasking.

The final strategy offered is more for maintenance of self. As I mentioned before, I believe relationships, sharing and listening, are instrumental for spiritual health. Many people speak of growth as an adult. In context, they likely are referring to emotional maturity and behavior. In my experience the most fruitful growth is that of the spirit. I believe that spiritual health begets that emotional maturity and behavior that is so calming and fulfilling. My goal is to continue spiritual growth through those relationships in my life. I try daily to connect with ***three people*** on a deeper level. It may be family or friends. Very frequently it is at the tables in the meetings of AA and NA. By deeper level I mean more than just asking how their day is, or how are the kids, or how's the new deck coming along. It may be difficult to share some things with family and friends. But I certainly feel safe and can trust my brothers and sisters in recovery. That is when the conversations can get deeper and more real, about love and honesty and acceptance and so many other aspects of life that addicts struggle with.

There is a wonderful analogy about recovery, a group of addicts being like a basketball team. The athletic trainer is your sponsor, on the sidelines with the coach, who is the higher power. All teammates are in recovery. The key is that no family members or friends can be on the team. They can be in the stands and cheer us on, but they will never know the game. Thus, my recommendation for these personal connections in recovery are those in the program. If a friend or family member is an addict, or in recovery, the relationship should still center around the family or friend aspect. You may go to meetings together and share, but sponsorship or other such connections should be avoided. The best explanation I have for the makeup of the team players is shared experience. The experiences of addiction, being at such a profound level as to cause changes in personality and behavior, are a strong bond when shared. Thus, the connection between addicts, the relationships, the sharing are all at a deeper level, allowing the addict to feel belonging, acceptance, and identification with a group.

Many victims of trauma participate in group therapy sessions regardless of any addiction sequelae. Cognitive behavioral therapy has once again been found to be very useful for these encounters. Once again, simplistically, the exercise being that of mindfulness, pulling the individual back to the moment, away from disturbing memories and emotions of the trauma, and then helping them to see and experience life without threat.

EPILOGUE

I am concerned when I hear addicts profess that they are sober for their loved one's sake, or the job, or to avoid legal issues. Recovery achieved by solely fear or solely reward requires tremendously more maintenance and vigilance than recovery that springs from the true love of self. While it is certainly true that many addicts have cleaned up for family or societal reasons, and any clean time is to be applauded, I feel this type of sobriety to be tenuous. I have sought here to identify and describe the deeper issues involved in the psychological origin and subsequent formation of an addict. Recovery for the self is pure and devoid of any extrinsic influence. I believe the root cause for addiction is self-hatred and feeling unlovable. Hypersensitivity and extreme empathy can manifest by nature or nurture, and at a very early age. These manifestations cause misunderstanding, feelings of being ostracized, and subsequently isolation.

Over these years of listening, sharing, and researching all aspects of addiction and alcoholism that I have encountered, I've discovered many important elements for successful recovery.

First, be honest with yourself. Write it down, jot notes in a journal or a piece of scratch paper at a meeting. Then revisit these notes in a day or two. But write down the "Aha!" moments. These brief yet powerful moments have been the guiding lights illuminating my path of recovery.

Second, focus on the moment. I try my best to stay in the present. We all need to make plans and hope and dream, but I do so with caution and vigilance. We have to have enough foresight to develop goals. Again, I try not to get too lofty or complex as this can lead to feelings of being overwhelmed. I focus on the three feet around me, trying to stay grounded and grateful. Gratitude begets happiness, not necessarily the other way around.

My third basic strategy is consistency. Consistency and repetition with honesty, and frequent grounding in the moment, have been my keys to defend against Slick. I have come to believe in the principals of the twelve-step programs of Alcoholics Anonymous and Narcotics Anonymous. They are simple programs, but they are not easy. I try to look at the brain as just a computer, and we need to do some repro-gramming. I believe the twelve steps has afforded me the code to do just that. This is where the message must be kept consistent and re-peated as much as possible. I find the meetings to be most helpful in this regard. Even a one-on-one phone conversation with a sponsor or another in the program can help. While the concept of a sponsor is not directly addressed in the Alcoholics Anonymous book, the principle has been found to be very helpful and robust.

Lastly is patience. Once again, not easy, but not complicated. The program works if you work it. I have heard that so many times. I wish I had listened sooner. It is simply the consistency and repetition that I speak of that is the work of recovery. Consistency in the following the steps. Repetition of the principles, the steps, the traditions and the promises of AA and NA. Another saying around the tables of the meetings is, "It takes as long as it takes." So, I try not to rush it. I don't feel that I've rushed it. But I have become one of those for-tunates that has seen the miracle in working the program. Just as the promises espouse.

As I have pursued recovery for the last twenty-five years, I failed repeatedly to achieve peace. Like many others, I sought an easier and quicker way to rid myself of addiction. Unfortunately, it took tremendous loss for me to finally reach the point of surrender. Just give up the fight. This is unacceptable in our culture, especially for a man. But it does not mean to quit. I try to use the word acceptance more. Accept that the conflicts will always be there. Accept that there will always be disagreements, differences of opinion. Accept that you cannot please everyone, and that there will always be those that don't like you no matter what you say or do. Most importantly, accept yourself, all of your imperfections and everything that makes you, you. After all, you are the one and only, the perfect you!

I am amazed at the similarities of stories of addicts. Some have been fortunate enough to have the psychological makeup to recognize the problem early on. Some stories end with a head marker. Most stories are in between these two. My story was riddled with temporary fixes, lip service, and going through the motions to satisfy the powers that be. As long as I held on to that hurtful belief that I was choosing to destroy my life, then I believed as our society professes, that we need to punish bad behavior. And if the bad behavior is caused by addiction, I have demonstrated that to punish an addict is exactly the opposite of what is needed to treat the disease. The worse the addict feels about himself, the more likely he is to use, to once again try to numb that spiritual pain.

My most sincere hope for anyone reading this book is peace. I found mine through gratitude and love. I believe you can too.

Hate the addiction, love the addict.

Godspeed.

BIBLIOGRAPHY

Alcoholics Anonymous. "The Big Book," fourth edition. 2001.

The Gifts of Imperfection; Brene Brown; 2010.

I Thought It Was Just Me; Brene Brown; 2007.

Your Owner's Manual; Burt Hotchkiss; 1992.

"Twelve Steps and Twelve Traditions"; AA World Services; 2002.

Pleasure Unwoven; Kevin McCauley; Hazelden Video Production; 2009.

Soul Murder, The Effects of Childhood Abuse and Deprivation; Leonhard Shengold, MD; 1991.

The Power of Now; Eckhart Tolle; 1999.

Kitchen Table Wisdom; Rachel Naomi Remen, MD; 1996.

A Return to Love; Marianne Williamson; 1996.

www.ingramcontent.com/pod-product-compliance
Lightning Source LLC
Chambersburg PA
CBHW060811260726
48660CB00002B/885